Weight Loss after childbirth

Tips for losing the baby Weight during postpartum Weight reduction

Linda A.shepherd

Table of content

Chapter 1

Weight loss after childbirth: Quick and healthy methods

It's plenty to cause many women to think about going on a diet or following a postpartum weight-loss plan and to question when they can begin.

The problem with the word 'dieting' is that it often indicates you need to restrict or exclude particular meals in order to lose weight, which isn't the case.

Not only is dieting not necessary for weight loss, but diets frequently result in lower intakes of vital vitamins, minerals, and nutrients. Your energy levels and postpartum recovery as well as the quantity and quality of your breast milk may be impacted by this.

Naturally, we don't want these for new mothers, especially those who are breastfeeding.Just as good nutrition is crucial throughout pregnancy, it's crucial afterward as well.

Furthermore, a lot of weight-loss programs are made to help you lose weight quickly, which might be unhealthy.
Of course, losing weight right away after delivery is typical. Additionally, you should anticipate losing a few more pounds in the week following birth.
and it will take time to shed it as well.
Rapid postpartum weight loss, defined as less than two pounds per week, is unhealthy, according to studies. Although it's crucial to finally reduce the excess weight you gained during pregnancy, you shouldn't rush or force the process.

Concentrating on healthy eating and portion control as opposed to dieting, further advice.

5 guidelines for weight loss after childbirth safety

That baby weight took time to gain, and it will take time to shed it as well.

Some offered advice on how to lose baby weight in a healthy manner.

1. Create attainable goals for weight loss

Knowing how long it often takes is the first step in putting yourself up for postpartum weight-loss success.

Most new mothers need six months to a year to reach their pre-pregnancy weight when they lose weight safely (approximately one pound per week).

In the first six weeks following delivery, half of that weight is usually lost. Women often drop the remaining weight at their own speed after that.

Use the advice below to stay on course as you go while being patient with your particular pace.

2. Consume balanced meals.

Focus on eating well-balanced meals, which include the following, rather than fad diets, which are frequently restricted and challenging to maintain:

You should have fruit and non-starchy vegetables on half of your plate.

Whole grains should make up one-fourth of your dish.

Lean protein should take up one-fourth of your plate.

a sprinkling of wholesome fats, such avocado, chia seeds, or olive oil.

Breastfeeding Section Collapse
breastfeeding is becoming more prevalent.
If you are nursing, you should reduce weight gradually. Rapid weight loss may cause you

to produce less milk. Losing roughly a pound and a half (670 grams) every week shouldn't have an impact on your health or ability to produce milk.

2. Consume balanced meals.

Focus on eating well-balanced meals, which include the following, rather than fad diets, which are frequently restricted and challenging to maintain:

You should have fruit and non-starchy vegetables on half of your plate.

Whole grains should make up one-fourth of your dish.

Lean protein should take up one-fourth of your plate.

a sprinkling of wholesome fats, such avocado, chia seeds, or olive oil.

Breastfeeding Section Collapse

breastfeeding is becoming more prevalent.

If you are nursing, you should reduce weight gradually. Rapid weight loss may cause you to produce less milk. Losing roughly a pound and a half (670 grams) every week shouldn't have an impact on your health or ability to produce milk.

Your body burns calories when breastfeeding, which aids with weight loss. You might be amazed at how much weight you naturally lose when breastfeeding if you're patient.

Collapse of Eat to Lose Weight The Eat to Lose Weight section has been increased.

You can safely lose weight by following these advice on eating healthy.

Don't miss any meals. Many new mothers neglect to eat when they have a baby. You will have less energy if you don't eat, and it won't help you lose weight.

Consume five to six modest meals and nutritious snacks throughout the day (rather than 3 larger meals).

consume breakfast. Even if you don't typically eat in the mornings, make breakfast a routine. You'll have more vigor to start the day and won't get exhausted later.

Speed up. You'll observe that it is simpler to recognize fullness when you eat slowly. While multitasking is alluring, focusing on your meal will reduce the likelihood that you may overindulge.

Try to incorporate fiber- and protein-rich meals in your snack selections to help you stay satisfied (such as raw bell pepper or carrot with bean dip, apple slices with peanut butter, or a slice of whole-wheat toast with hard-boiled egg). Take at least 12 cups of liquid daily.

can hinder your efforts to lose weight. Products with artificial sweeteners should be avoided.

Instead of fruit juice, use the whole fruit. Fruit juices should be consumed sparingly because they provide additional calories. Whole fruits provide you with vitamins, nutrients, and more fiber, which makes you feel satisfied on fewer calories.

Choose baked or broiled cuisine over fried options.
Limit sugar, saturated fat, and sweets.

Taking care of a newborn, settling into a new routine, and recovering after childbirth can be stressful. That is a lot.

After birth, it's crucial to get back to a healthy weight, especially if you want to have another child in the future.
We'll go through some proven techniques to assist you in getting to a healthy postpartum weight so you can embrace parenthood with enthusiasm.

How much is "baby weight"?
Here is some background information on "baby weight," why it occurs during pregnancy, and why it won't be necessary once the kid is born.

The Centers for Disease Control and Prevention (CDC) advises healthy-weight women who are expecting one child should gain 25–35 pounds (11.5–16 kg) during pregnancy.
Different weight-gain recommendations are made for expecting women who are underweight, overweight, or carrying multiple kids. To find out your specific recommended weight gain, use the interactive calculators at the Institute of Medicine/National Academies.

Depending on your particular needs, your healthcare experts can provide different advice.

Pregnancy weight gain includes the following Source:
infant placenta
Breast tissue, blood, uterine enlargement, and amniotic fluid
excess fat reserves

The excess fat serves as a source of energy during breastfeeding and childbirth. However, gaining too much weight might lead to having too much fat. This is what is typically referred to as "baby weight," and it happens frequently.

Over half of all pregnant women acquire more weight during pregnancy than is advised.

The following are the effects of carrying some of this additional weight after giving birth:

greater risk of diabetes and heart disease due to being overweight
problems are more likely to occur during pregnancy
Women with gestational diabetes face greater health risks.
Evidence-based weight loss advice is provided in the list that follows.
Advice for reducing pregnancy weight

1. Make realistic goals.
Contrary to what publications and celebrity accounts would have you believe, postpartum weight loss takes time.

According to a 2015 study, 75% of women had gained more weight a year after giving birth than they had before becoming pregnant. At one year, 25% of these women had maintained 20 additional pounds, and 47% had gained at least 10 pounds.

It is reasonable to anticipate that over the following one to two years, you could shed about 10 pounds, depending on how much weight you put on during pregnancy (4.5 kg). If you put on extra weight, you might discover that you're a few pounds heavier than you were before being pregnant.

2. Avoid crash dieting
Crash diets are very low calorie diets that are designed to help you lose a significant amount of weight as quickly as possible.

Your body needs a healthy diet to heal and recuperate after childbirth. Additionally, breastfeeding increases your calorie needs.

Low calorie diets are typically deficient in essential nutrients and will probably make you feel lethargic. This is the exact opposite of what you need when caring for a newborn and are probably exhausted.

If your weight is constant right now, cutting 500 calories from your daily consumption will result in a safe loss of 1.1 pounds (0.5 kg) per week.

A lady who consumes 2,000 calories per day, for instance, might eat 300 fewer calories and burn an additional 200 calories through activity, for a total decrease of 500 calories.

3. If you are able, breastfeed.
Breastfeeding is advised by the American Academy of Pediatrics (AAP), the CDC, and the World Health Organization (WHO)Trusted Source. There are numerous advantages for both you and your baby when you breastfeed during the first six months of life (or much longer):

Nutrition: breast milk supplies all the nutrients a baby needs to grow and thrive in the first six months of life.
strengthens the infant's immune system Additionally, essential antibodies found in breast milk help your infant fight off infections and viruses.
reduces the risk of disease in infants: Babies who are breastfed have a lower risk of gastrointestinal infections, asthma, obesity, type 1 diabetes, respiratory disease, ear infections, and sudden infant death syndrome (SIDS).

Reduces the mother's risk of illness: Breastfeeding mothers are less likely to have ovarian, breast, or high blood pressure, type 2 diabetes, high cholesterol, or high blood pressure.

Additionally, studies have shown that breastfeeding might help you lose weight after giving birth.

However, during the first three months of nursing, you could not lose any weight or even put on a little. Due to higher calorie requirements and intake as well as decreased physical activity when lactating, this is the case.

4. Keep an eye on your caloric intake

We are aware that not everyone should track calories. However, if you find that eating intuitively isn't working for you, tracking your calories can help you figure out how much you're consuming and where any potential problem areas in your diet are.

It can also assist you in ensuring that you consume enough calories to give you the nutrition and energy you require.

This is possible by:
using a mobile calorie counting software, keeping a food journal, and taking pictures of your meals to help you remember what you've eaten
discussing your daily caloric intake with a pal who is also keeping track of their intake to maintain accountability
You can minimize your portion sizes and make healthier food choices by using these strategies, which will aid in weight loss.

5. Take in fiber-rich foods
Get those wholesome grains and vegetables on your shopping list right away. It has been demonstrated that consuming meals high in fiber can aid in weight loss.
For instance, over 345 individuals discovered that adding 4 grams of fiber to what participants were already eating before

the study resulted in an additional average weight loss of 3 1/4 pounds over the course of six months.

According to science, soluble fiber foods (like these!) may also help you feel fuller for longer by slowing down digestion and lowering hunger hormone levels.

Although the overall findings of research are conflicting, these impacts on digestion might aid in calorie restriction.

6. Stock up on protein-rich foods
According to studies reported in the American Journal of Clinical Nutrition, including protein in your diet can increase metabolism, lower appetite, and help you consume less calories.
Protein, compared to other nutrients, has a stronger "thermic" effect, according to studies. This indicates that it requires more energy for the body to digest than other

forms of food, resulting in more calories being burned.

Furthermore, ResearchTrusted Source demonstrates that protein can reduce appetite by lowering ghrelin and raising the hormones that promote fullness, GLP and GLP-1. Less hormones of hunger equals less rage!

Suitable sources of protein include:

Low mercury seafood, lean meats, eggs, beans, nuts, and seeds
dairy
Check out these lightweight, high-protein snacks you can carry with you.
7. Keep wholesome snacks close by
What you eat can be greatly influenced by the meals that are available to you. A healthy substitute is ideal when you're browsing the pantry for something to snack on.

You may make sure you have something on hand when the mood strikes by stocking up on healthy snacks. Following are some to have on hand:

hummus, sliced vegetables, mixed nuts, and dried fruit

String cheese, handmade granola, air-popped popcorn, spiced nuts, and seaweed snacks

Simply leaving fruit out on the counter has been linked to a lower body mass index,Comparative research also revealed that keeping unhealthy items out on the counter is linked to an increase in weight. Keep processed meals and sweets away from the kitchen, or better yet, keep them outside the house.

We adore these nutritious snack suggestions for the workplace, pantry, and other locations.

Chapter 2

foods to stay away from while nursing

To make sure you're getting everything you need, try to eat the following things every day:

foods high in protein. Aim for a minimum of three servings per day, which can include tofu, meat, lentils, yogurt, nut butter, and cheese.
whole grains. To stay energized, you should consume three or more servings of complex carbohydrates with fiber each day, such as oatmeal, brown rice, and barley.
Fruits and vegetables. Eat four to five servings of vegetables per day, focusing on leafy green and yellow vegetables.
fattening foods. Attempt to consume as much as you did while pregnant. Healthy

fats can be found in avocados, low-mercury seafood, nuts, and seeds and should be included in your diet.

You must also remember to consume certain nutrients, like as

Calcium. You require between 1,000 and 1,500 milligrams, and it's crucial to consume enough because breastfeeding depletes your calcium stores. Cheese, yogurt, milk, collard greens, sardines, tofu, and chia seeds are all excellent sources.

Iron. An iron-rich diet, such as beef, chicken, eggs, beans, or fortified cereal, should be consumed in one or more servings per day.

C vitamin. This crucial antioxidant is abundant in berries, bell peppers, citrus, broccoli, and other fruits and vegetables.

Omega-3s. To encourage baby's brain development, aim to consume two to three servings of foods containing omega-3 fatty acids per week. That is a minimum of 8 ounces every week of wild salmon and sardines, which are low in mercury, as well as eggs that have been supplemented with DHA.

Choline. Your daily requirements really rise from 450 to 550 mg after giving birth. This essential nutrient helps your baby's brain development when you're nursing.

Continue taking your prenatal vitamin daily while breastfeeding even after the baby is born to cover all your bases.

For a quick snack, I highly suggest the new Milk Dust Lactation bars! They are delicious, loaded with protein, low in sugar, and packed with herbs that will help you have more children.

Fresh berries, cucumber slices, hummus, and apple slices with one tablespoon of peanut butter are all served with a handful of nuts.

Lunch: a substantial salad with roasted sweet potatoes, lettuce, tomatoes, cilantro, and chickpeas.

Add salt, pepper, and a dab of balsamic vinegar on the top.

Add a small amount of goat cheese or feta cheese on top.

If you have some sliced fruit, include it as well!

Snack: Roasted vegetables, half-baked sweet potato, turkey slices on top of cucumbers with mustard, and one slice of avocado toast on sprouted bread.

Evening options include turkey chili, baked salmon with basmati rice, lightened-up nachos (recipe in the program), sheet pan steak and vegetables, or another sizable salad with rotisserie chicken sliced in.

Lunch: a substantial salad with roasted sweet potatoes, lettuce, tomatoes, cilantro, and chickpeas.

Add salt, pepper, and a dab of balsamic vinegar on the top.

Add a small amount of goat cheese or feta cheese on top.
If you have some sliced fruit, include it as well!

Snack: Roasted vegetables, half-baked sweet potato, turkey slices on top of cucumbers with mustard, and one slice of avocado toast on sprouted bread.

Evening options include turkey chili, baked salmon with basmati rice, lightened-up nachos (recipe in the program), sheet pan steak and vegetables, or another sizable salad with rotisserie chicken sliced in.

In contrast to what you would believe, if you have a meal plan, you can cook less rather than more. That is, of course, assuming that your meal plan emphasizes quick and simple meals, includes some meal preparation, includes crockpot meals, and so on. No one has time for elaborate 3-course dinners, thus none of them do it.

Also, you won't have to waste time and effort dragging your children on yet another grocery store trip because you were looking up a recipe on Pinterest and discovered you were missing one or more of the required ingredients. You may even be able to get your goods online with a meal plan, which would spare you from ever having to visit another corona-infested grocery store. supermarket from the inside!

Sounds challenging? If you have the proper meal plan, it isn't. The appropriate strategy will not only give you the nutrition you need for yourself and your child, but it will also prevent you from overeating or undereating, which are both fairly prevalent in breastfeeding mothers.

Chapter 3

Health advantages of postpartum exercise

Exercise after giving birth has a wealth of advantages for your health as well as for your mood and stress levels. Exercise not only promotes physical healing but also gives you a chance to center yourself and focus on you, which may feel a little difficult now that you are taking care of a small child. "Postpartum exercise gives moms back that sensation of being in control, It greatly reduces stress and provides new mothers something on which to fully concentrate.

Regular exercise after childbirth gives both physical and mental power a significant boost. "You recently went through a lot of changes; things have changed. Exercise aids in internal healing.

Postnatal exercise can result in weight loss, increased strength (carrying a baby around all the time is no joke), better sleep, and more balanced hormones—essential after nine months of ups and downs—in addition to the many psychological and emotional advantages.

First things first: Ask your doctor before beginning a postpartum workout regimen. It typically varies, but many doctors advise waiting six to eight weeks following delivery before beginning any kind of activity. Complications in pregnancy or labor can cause some women to be delayed by a few extra weeks. For instance, a mother who gave birth vaginally will probably have a different chronology than one who gave birth via cesarean. Others could even be able to start exercising earlier than six weeks.

When it's time to start exercising again,The muscle in your bodyAfter giving birth, your memory will start working, making it easier for you to get back into it. Despite this, you should still give your body some time to rest.

Never overexert yourself after having a kid. The key is patience.

Working with your doctor to determine the precise timing that is best for you and your health is essential, regardless of the situation. Every mom is different, and it's vital to pay attention to pressures the body may experience post-pregnancy." A doctor will be able to look for signs of diastasis recti (the separation of the abdominal muscles) and offer the right physical therapy to treat it or any other postpartum complications.
It's crucial to keep your expectations in check before you start exercising again. You won't immediately regain your former strength because of the changes to your physique. Start with easy, practical exercises that you may advance from.

solitary-arm rows
They can be carried out using a dumbbell, resistance band, or cable. Start with a little weight, ideally between 2 and 5 pounds.

Maintain a square posture. Stand up straight if you're using a cable or band. When using a dumbbell, keep your knees open and gently hunch at the waist. Pull back the arm while holding the while engaging your core.weight until your elbow by the side of your body forms a 90-degree angle. Before alternating arms, retract and repeat for 10 times. This exercises your triceps, biceps, and upper back.

Rotations of wall planks
For those with diastasis recti or anyone easing back into core activity (for example, if you're recovering from a c-section), this postpartum exercise is perfect. Choose a solid wall, face it, and place your feet about two feet from the wall. You should be in a standing plank position with your forearms resting against the wall. Retract your shoulders as you slowly twist your torso out to create a wall-based side plank position. Before going back to the beginning position

and switching sides, hold for two counts. On each side, repeat for 10 times. This is excellent for the upper body and some mild core exercise.

Raised push-ups to wall push-ups
As with the Wall Plank Rotations, begin in the same place. Do a push-up plank position with your hands up against the wall. Focus on keeping your body in a straight line while maintaining a neutral spine and engaging your core. Lower your body toward the wall while bending your arms like you would for a push-up. Back away and straighten your spine.

arms. When your upper body strength gradually improves, you can progress to higher push-ups (push-ups with your feet on a bench or chair). This exercises your chest, biceps, and triceps.

breathing with the diaphragm
Start out in a supine (backwards) position with your legs straight out and your arms at

your sides. Fill your tummy up by inhaling. After that, press your lower back against the ground while completely exhaling. It's a relaxing postpartum ab workout that's classy.

Cat/Cows
Start on all fours, stacking your shoulders over your hands and your feet.arms. When your upper body strength gradually improves, you can progress to higher push-ups (push-ups with your feet on a bench or chair). This exercises your chest, biceps, and triceps.

breathing with the diaphragm
Start out in a supine (backwards) position with your legs straight out and your arms at your sides. Fill your tummy up by inhaling. After that, press your lower back against the ground while completely exhaling. It's a relaxing postpartum ab workout that's classy.

Supine Leg Lifts
Begin in a supine position with your lower back pressed into the ground. Bring the legs straight into the air to create a 90-degree angle from your waist. Inhale and slowly lower your legs down as far as you can. Feel free to lower one leg at a time, and bend your knee as a modification. Exhale and bring the leg back up. Perform 10 reps on each side. This helps strengthen deep pelvic floor muscles and the transverse abdominal muscles

Spine leg lift
With your legs at a 90-degree angle, sit against a wall. Hold for 30 seconds with your back flush against the wall. After another 30 seconds of holding, let go and rest. Then do it five more times. Your core and quads will be worked.

Dead bugs
Start in a supine position with your arms and legs fully extended. While you exhale,

lower your left leg and arm (your arm should go back toward your head, not your feet). Raise both after exhaling. On the right side, repeat. Your oblique muscles are worked by this.

Wall sits

With your legs at a 90-degree angle, sit against a wall. Hold for 30 seconds with your back flush against the wall. After another 30 seconds of holding, let go and rest. Then do it five more times. Your core and quads will be worked.

Quadruped leg lift

Start on all fours with your hips just above your knees, your shoulders directly above your hands. Using your glutes and leg muscles, straighten one leg out behind you. Hold for a short while, then go back to where you were at the beginning and flip sides. On each side, repeat for 10 times. This exercises your hamstrings, glutes, and core.

Your physique has changed since then! Remember that it will be challenging to find time to workout in addition to your body feeling unusual and occasionally weak before you get back into your fitness regimen. That's okay. Young mothers should be patient with themselves.

Don't give up if it takes longer to get back into exercising or to feel at ease exercising again, she advises. Don't push yourself too hard too soon; pay attention to your body. She continues by saying that doing so could lead to further stress, which would only cause you to fall behind psychologically and physically.

The outcome of your pregnancy and delivery will determine when you can resume exercising safely. You can begin modest exercise as soon as a few days after giving birth if you had an easy pregnancy and regular vaginal delivery. If youYour body probably needs additional time if you had a difficult pregnancy or had a cesarean section. You can learn when you can resume exercising from your doctor

Moreover, light exercise needs to receive some attention. It may be alluring to try to take on too much too soon, especially if you miss your prior exercise regimen.

Regardless of your level of fitness before becoming pregnant, starting slowly and following your body's cues. "During pregnancy, there are structural and hormonal changes that overdoing it after giving birth can cause joint pain, injury, and urinary or fecal leakages. Pregnancy symptoms don't just go away once the baby is delivered.

Before going for a run or doing an HIIT workout, choose low-impact exercises like walking or postpartum exercises to gradually ease into exercise. Also, as you gradually raise the difficulty of your workouts over time, pay attention to your body's signals and stop right away if you experience any pain. Most importantly, make sure your fitness goals are reasonable. Keep in mind that, in addition to regaining strength, boosting your general health is important if you're new to exercising and trying to shed some baby weight.

Building muscle and maintaining cardiovascular health require time. Even if you already exercise frequently, you still need to be patient as your body heals.

Here are some suggestions for exercising while nursing:

Drink a lot of water.

Do wear an appropriate-fitting, supportive bra (not too tight, but not too loose)

Do progressively up your degree of activity.

Don't work out while you have large breasts (breastfeed or pump before a workout)

Avoid overdoing it since stress and exhaustion can decrease your milk production and raise your chance of developing a breast infection.

Chapter 4

Items to avoid eating when nursing

If you are what you consume, then your breastfeeding child must also be. They should only receive the best nutrients, therefore stay away from potentially harmful items. But because there is so much conflicting information available, breastfeeding parents frequently swear off entire food categories out of fear.

Good news: There are fewer foods to avoid when breastfeeding than you might have believed. Why? Considering that your milk-producing cells and mammary glands assist control how the majority of what you consume actually makes its way to your kid through your milk.

Before you start cutting things out of your diet while you're breastfeeding, read on to learn the verdict on things like alcohol, caffeine, and other items that were off-limits during pregnancy.

By the time a baby begins nursing, they are used to the tastes that their parents consume. According to science, eating a wide variety of meals during pregnancy alters the amniotic fluid's flavor and smell, which the baby is exposed to and is smelling in utero. "And breastfeeding is basically the next phase after conception."enters the breast milk from the amniotic fluid.

In fact, newborns are drawn to some substances that parents opt to avoid during breastfeeding, such as spices and hot meals. Where moms who were nursing their infants were given a garlic pill while others received a placebo. The babies drank more milk flavored with garlic than milk without garlic, as well as nursing for a longer period of time.

If they believe there is a link between what they ate and their child's behavior—gassy, irritable, etc.—parents frequently restrict their diet. Even while the cause-and-effect relationship might appear to be sufficient.

"I would need to see problems with the stools being abnormal in order to declare with certainty that a newborn had something that was milk-related. It is quite uncommon for a baby to have a condition that would prevent the mother from breastfeeding."

Alcohol Evaluation:
Moderate Use is Safe
The laws regarding alcohol are altered once your child is born! Drinking the equivalent of a 12-ounce beer, a 4-ounce glass of wine, or one ounce of hard liquor once or twice a week is safe, say specialists. The amount of alcohol that does enter into breast milk is usually quite little.

Caffeine is Safe in Moderation

Drinking coffee, tea, and caffeinated sodas in moderation is acceptable during breastfeeding. Less than 1% of the caffeine consumed by the mother normally finds its way into the breast milk. Also, there is little to no caffeine found in the baby's urine if you only consume three cups of coffee throughout the day.

Consider reducing your intake or delaying reintroducing coffee until your child is older, though, if you notice that your baby becomes fussier or angrier when you consume too much caffeine (often more than five caffeinated beverages per day).

According to studies, most infants' sleep patterns weren't negatively impacted by a breastfeeding parent's caffeine usage by the time they were three to six months old.

According to the available clinical evidence, I encourage patients to wait until their child is at least three months old before reintroducing caffeine to their diet, and then to keep an eye out for any signs of discomfort or restlessness in the child.

If you're a mom who works outside the home, I advise you to always label any milk you pump after consuming caffeine so the baby doesn't drink it immediately before naptime or night.

Caffeine is naturally found in coffee, tea, chocolate, and soda, but it is also present in large quantities in foods and drinks that have coffee- or chocolate-flavored flavors. If your baby is especially sensitive to caffeine, keep in mind that even decaffeinated coffee contains some of it.

Verdict on Sushi: Safe with Moderation
You can relax knowing that sushi that doesn't contain high-mercury seafood is okay to eat while nursing if you've been holding out for 40 weeks. This results from the Listeria bacteria,

which, is present in undercooked food, is not easily transmitted through breast milk.

The maximum amount of low-mercury fish that should be consumed in a week is two to three servings (a maximum of twelve ounces), if you decide to eat one of these low-mercury sushi options while nursing. Salmon, flounder, tilapia, trout, pollock, and catfish are examples of fish that typically have low mercury concentrations.

Judgment on High-Mercury Fish: Avoid
Fish can be a nutrient-dense part of your diet when prepared healthfully, like by baking or broiling. However because of a variety of variables,
Moreover, the majority of fish and other seafood contain harmful toxins, including mercury. Mercury may build up in the body and quickly reach harmful amounts. Elevated mercury levels primarily impact the central nervous system and result in neurological defects.

For this reason, high-mercury foods have been advised against by the US Food and Drug Administration (FDA), Environmental Protection Agency (EPA), and World Health Organization (WHO). There are also particular recommendations set forth by the EPA for healthy adults because mercury is one of the top ten substances of significant public health concern, according to the WHO.based on gender and weight.

Tuna, shark, swordfish, mackerel, and tilefish are all on the list of foods to stay away from since they frequently contain higher levels of mercury and should always be avoided when nursing.

Most breastfeeding mothers can eat a variety of foods without their newborns being harmed. Yet each circumstance is unique. See your baby's doctor to determine whether your diet or something else may be to blame if you notice that your baby becomes fussy, restless, or gassy after you consume a certain meal.

mothers who breastfeed include:

Avoid consuming the following mercury-rich fish species:

Shark Swordfish King Mackerel
Ruddy marlin orange
Tilefish from the Gulf of Mexico that are
bigeye tuna
But, provided you limit your intake and select low-mercury fish and seafood, you can consume fish while nursing. In fact, eating 8 to 12 ounces of low-mercury fish each week is advised for breastfeeding mothers as it is a wonderful source of DHA and EPA, two omega-3 fatty acids that are hard to get in other meals.

Moreover, you can have raw fish while nursing! Contrary to pregnancy, seared tuna, poke, and sushi are not to be avoided.

It's best to avoid drinking any alcohol while nursing, however it's acceptable to indulge sometimes if you:

Timing is everything. If at all possible, breastfeed your child right away before drinking (or pump breast milk). Wait at least two hours before nursing after consuming alcohol. Before that waiting period expires, if your breasts are full, you can pump and dispense your breast milk. Feed your infant already expressed breast milk if they need to eat before the two hours are up.
Consider personal factors that may affect blood alcohol content. They include your weight and whether you've eaten anything.
Drink responsibly. The hold-up time is
Unless you have an older infant who doesn't nurse as regularly, it's challenging to consume more than one drink responsibly. This waiting period is crucial because the same amount of alcohol that enters your circulation also enters your breast milk.

Herbs: Certain herbal products, including some herbal teas, aren't thought to be suitable for nursing mothers. Before taking any herbs, consult with your doctor because they can be very potent. Moreover, some herbs can reduce your milk production.

Chocolate: Consuming too much could overwhelm your child. But the sums involved are considerable. You can indulge in a few chocolate treats.
perhaps a chocolate cake slice. Yet if you consume a lot of chocolate, theobromine, a stimulant, can have a similar effect on your child as caffeine does.

White chocolate contains no theobromine, but dark chocolate contains more theobromine than milk chocolate (the ingredient is in the cocoa solids). Another reason not to overindulge is the presence of caffeine in chocolate.

It is doable. See your baby's doctor if it appears that an item in your diet is causing a reaction. A dietary intolerance might be the cause, or it might be something else.

An allergy is an immunological reaction, whereas an intolerance is a digestive problem. Food intolerance symptoms include:
Fussiness
Congestion
Rash
Vomiting
Bloody diarrhea
The two most common causes of food intolerances in infancy are:

If your kid has a cow's milk protein intolerance, you should keep them away from foods that contain milk, milk products, casein, whey, or sodium caseinate.
If your kid has soy protein intolerance, stay away from all soy products such tofu,

tempeh, tamari, soy sauce, soy milk, miso, and edamame.

Even if you consume allergenic foods like peanuts, fish, shellfish, and eggs, your breast milk is very unlikely to cause an allergic reaction in your kid.

If your child experiences allergy symptoms like eczema or a rash, runny nose, sneezing, coughing, red and watery eyes, vomiting, or diarrhea, it's possible that these symptoms are brought on by things they frequently come into contact with like soap, pet dander, dust, pollen, or other allergens.
When babies begin eating solids, the meals they consume.

Rarely, a newborn may develop an allergy to foods that their mother ate, such as cow's milk protein. Consult with your baby's doctor to determine whether you should be concerned about a reaction to allergenic foods you consume. A breastfed infant with a food allergy can only be managed by careful dietary abstinence.

However, you should consult your nursing baby's doctor if you notice that they become fussy, gassy, or restless after you eat a certain food. They might advise you to cut the meal out of your diet for at least three weeks before reintroducing it to determine if the effects persist.